Cheers! To Good Health
Getting Fit, Living Fearless, Looking Fabulous

Table of Contents

My Story: How It All Started

When I started my journey, I didn't realize it would turn into a movement. God always makes something good out of a hurt person. And hurt I was. I was in a dark space in my life. To be honest, my whole life up until now has been dark. I have been holding onto a lot of pain and sorrow, from when I was a child. I had 3 children in sorrow, got married in sorrow. I know that these should have been some of the best times of my life. After all, they were moments of celebration. But once we stop celebrating, the sadness always seemed to be there waiting. Was it stealing my joy, or was I sacrificing it for my sadness? I don't know.

What I do know is that I didn't start living my life until Spring of 2014. I feel like a new person, not just on the outside but the inside. I had a spiritual awakening. You see, when you change what you put in your body, you actually help change your thoughts as well. The first decision I made was to cut out beef, pork, and soda. The reason why I made these changes started when I checked my blood pressure at one of those self-service deals. The machine translated that I needed to consult my doctor immediately. The interesting thing is that I instantly noticed a difference in my body.

I dropped 20 pounds and my thoughts became clearer. I started juicing and eating more raw foods. Did you know the junk you put in your body affects the way you think and act? Did you know that more than half the population has parasites living in their bodies? I did a parasite cleanse for 7 days to make sure I got all those creatures out of my body. And yes, I had them in my body. They drain all your energy, and cause your stomach to always feel and look blown out. What's more, parasites can kill you. They literally suck the life out of you. I remember during that cleanse on day 4 I felt something moving around my abdomen. It was as if what I was doing was irritating the parasites. The next day something that looked like a snake, a very long snake dropped as I was helping myself in the toilet. You should be doing a parasite cleanse 4 times a year, once in every season.

There is no proven way to avoid them, because they are all over. Unless you live in a bubble, you have probably been exposed to some type of parasite. I learned the key to being and staying healthy is to pay close attention to your body. You shouldn't feel tired and fatigued all the time. Watch what you put in your mouth and whose hands handle what you put in your mouth. Fast food or dining out should only be done on special occasions -not every day, and not more than once per day. That's if you want to live a long full life. Changes like that will make a big difference in the way your body feels. Stop dieting.

The most important factor you need to consider is the reason why you want to lose weight. Is it to look good or is it to feel good. For me it was to feel better. I slept all the time because I always felt really tired, angry, and depressed. Most of my overweight was from stress eating. I used to be one of those people who say, "you only live once, so why not eat what you want".

The truth is that no one can eat what they want, when they want and live a long healthy life- no one. We all want to eat junk food. Junk Food is highly addictive and those parasites love junk food. Don't get me wrong; I still have a chip or two. They don't taste the same though. Over time, your taste buds will adjust to healthier food. When I do drink juices, I have to add water because it's too much for my taste buds. You can train your body to do whatever you want it to do. Remember that most people do not realize that before you can change your body, you need to change your mindset first. Stop eating in bed or while lying down. I'm sure you have heard that before. Binge eating diets was a big problem of mine. A diet is just that - a diet. As soon as you stop dieting, you're going to gain the weight back. This book is about lifestyle changes. You must be willing to exercise at least 4 times a week for maintenance and to keep your body toned. During this journey I eat some of the things I like.

One I started paying close attention to the food I ate; I soon found that I no longer had the craving for most of the food I loved.

The holistic nature of weight loss

It is important to keep in mind that food is for nourishment. We have taken eating to a whole different level. It is like an event for some people, and once they do sit down to eat, they eat too much. This is not intended to put anyone down or to make them feel bad about themselves. The point here is to help you understand why you're over weight. After reading this book you will make up your mind that you will no longer tolerate this type of behavior from yourself. We were not created to be unhealthy, unhappy and whatever else that's going on in your life. Close your eyes for 1 minute and think about the people you love. How much do you love them? That's how much you should want to change. In order for your outside to change, your inside has to start the change. Look in the mirror - get mad, happy or whatever emotion you need to feel to get you going. I'm going to be hard on you because I want good health for you, even if you don't want it. Stop giving up so easily. How many times have you started a "diet" and gave up before you actually saw the results you were seeking? Well, so have I; that's why I can truly say it starts from within. In this book, I plan to cover blood types, the use of herbs, the importance of raw foods vs. cooked foods.

Evaluate your life

What do your daily activities look like? How much breathing, sweating are you doing? Stop being too busy for yourself. If working out is too intense for you right now, start with yoga. Spend at least 30-45 minutes a day on your body. This goes back to your why? Why are you reading this book right now? Why do you want to lose weight? For me it's deeper than a dress size; I want to live long and strong. I don't want to spend my life in a doctor's office. Good health starts with the mind; how you feel is in your mind. It has nothing to do with your body. The human body is led by the tongue and the mind. We have to learn how to control our thoughts. Negative thoughts are going to always try to creep in. And that's when you should be full armed with weapons such as self affirmations. When something negative comes your way, start speaking your personal affirmations. Don't rely on anyone else to lift you up but yourself and God. Stop giving things and people those types of responsibilities. So, how can you deal with negative thoughts? We will learn all that in a subsequent chapter but for now, let me give you some more information about me and the life that described who I was an how I actually changed.

Who I was and How I changed

Here's some personal info about me - not only was I overweight, but I was also a smoker; I had been a smoker for 20 years although I didn't smoke while I was pregnant with my children. Other than that, I smoked every day until now...My children have never lived in a smoke-free home up until now. I give detox credit for most of my success in weight loss and in stopping smoking. Your body's releasing all the harmful toxins. Toxins in the body cause us to do things that we as humans wouldn't do. Be mindful of the things you put in your body from the word go. We all want to lose weight without exercise but that's not possible and even if you do, you still have to tone your body and maintain the weight loss. My program is not about carb and calorie counting. We can't totally deprive ourselves of the things we like. So the key is to balance. Always think balance when you're eating and preparing meals. You can eat whatever you want to eat; just not a lot and not every day. My mindset in this process was that I wanted to get into a size 12 and I stayed focused on that. That meant giving up on some foods simply because I wanted to get into that size.

How to get started

Create a vision of yourself- what's your goal weight? What size are you now in and what size do you want to be? Apple cider vinegar and honey is a great natural resource for weight loss. This journey has been long. I say that because your weight loss journey doesn't start when you lose your first pound - it starts when you realize a change needs to be made concerning your weight. Some people struggle with weight loss before they can actually make some real changes. I have now started eating my favorite foods and no longer count calories. I always keep balance in perspective; I can eat that piece of cake if I go to the gym and be willing to work it off. One should be in tune with their chakra, all 7. You should strive towards ensuring that you balance these chakras since states of imbalance often result to numerous complications including stress. As we all know, stress largely contributes to weight gain because of the effect of the stress hormone cortisol (we will talk about that later). Before we start this weight loss journey, we must first learn why we are overweight. Food can be an addiction, just like gambling, smoking, and drinking. If you don't control or master your addiction, then you will soon get back to the same condition of obesity once stress is applied. It goes back to what I stated earlier in the book - it's a mental thing. We have to control our thoughts in the mind. Balance is key to a successful journey - whatever that journey may be.

What's your why? Why do want to lose weight?

What's Your Ideal Body Weight Range?

If you are trying to lose weight, the first question you should probably address is your ideal weight for your age and height. To determine your ideal weight, you should consider several factors, including your age, bone density, sex, height, and muscle fat ratio. Some health professionals recommend calculating your BMI (Body Mass Index) as the best way to determine whether your body weight is ideal. Others argue that the process is faulty and that it does not account for muscle mass, and are instead in favor of waist hip ratio. Different people have different ideal body weights. If you compare yourself to friends or family, you may end up aiming too high if you are surrounded by overweight or obese people. On the other hand, you may end up aiming too low if everyone around you looks like a fashion model. The levels of obesity and overweight in one country vary greatly from those in another country. For example, the number of obese and overweight people in the UK or USA is much higher than in Holland. Therefore, if all a Dutch person did was to compare him/herself to an American, he would basically aim for a lower ideal weight.

Your body mass index is your weight in relation to your height.

BMI metric units are calculated by dividing your weight in kilograms by your height in meters squared. For example, if you have a height of 1.8m and weigh 80kgs, your BMI is 80/3.24 (3.24 is the square of 1.8), which totals to 24.69.

Imperial units are calculated as follows:

(Your weight in pounds x 703) / The square of your height in inches

For example: if you weigh 190 pounds and are 6ft in height; then your BMI= (190x703)/5184, which is 25.76

Amidst the various disagreements, health professionals around the world agree that people with a BMI 18.5 and below are underweight, and that a BMI range of between 18.5 & 25 is ideal. If you have a BMI of between 25 & 30 you are considered overweight, while if you have a BMI of over 30 you are considered obese. You can use an online calculator to determine your BMI, such as this one.

So, if you find you are overweight based on your BMI, you need to take measures to lose the excess weight to get your body to an ideal weight for your height. Obviously, with all the fad diets crushing people's dreams of ever losing their weight, you need to settle for a sustainable weight loss regime if you really want to lose weight and keep it off. You don't want to lose over 10 pounds in 2 weeks then gain all that and some more within the next few months. However, before you can start your weight loss journey, it is perhaps important to first understand why you are overweight or obese in the first place. Like I said, knowing your why can be the first step to sustainable weight loss since you can help remedy the problem from its root. Let's take a look at some reasons why you could be overweight or obese.

>Failing to get enough sleep: If you don't get enough sleep, you are likely to crave for comfort foods and even have unbalanced hormone levels. Actually, the levels of the hormone cortisol are often high when you are not getting enough sleep. Failing to have enough sleep also causes fluctuations of the hunger hormone ghrelin and leptin resulting to heightened levels of hunger.

>Eating out too often: Before I started my weight loss journey, I felt "proud" of eating out. However, I was actually eating more calories than necessary because I felt obliged to eat all the food I was served. Many are the times when I was eating unhealthy foods like French fries, pizza and other unhealthy foods.

>Serving larger proportions of foods: If you feel "justified" to eat more food, you need to take action because you are constantly taking more calories than your body needs resulting to a calorie surplus, which clearly results to weight increase.

>Not watching what you drink: If you are constantly taking soft drinks and other energy drinks, you can bet that you are adding more calories to your body. Your morning cup of coffee e.g. iced Cappuccino could have over 200 calories, over 10 grams of fat and over 50 grams of sodium. If you top this on an already full stomach, you will definitely add weight because of calorie surplus. So if you are very accustomed to sugary drinks, you should start taking action now.

>Stress: Stress causes an increase in the levels of the stress hormone cortisol, which results to drastic storage of fat. With high levels of cortisol, the body reduces metabolism to conserve energy so that it can have enough for the fight and flight response. This results to storage of more fat when you don't find avenues for using the stored energy.

>Failing to see the "hidden" calories: When I first started taking action on my weight, I started by drastically reducing my intake of sugary stuff. Although this was a step in the right direction, I didn't realize that I still had a lot to do in cutting down my intake of unhealthy foods. One such food was unhealthy fat. I was still taking the wrong kinds of fats that were making it harder for me to lose weight. Besides, some of these fats were putting my health at risk of cardiovascular problems. You don't have to learn the hard way; you should also start taking healthy fats and in low quantities. Frying food doesn't mean that it should be all glittery! Eat more healthy fats like avocado, olive oil and coconut oil.

When I knew all that, I took action using a strategy that probably everyone who has lost weight in a healthy way could associate with. I will show you my secret to sustainable weight loss, which I can sum in simple steps namely:

#1: Detoxify

#2: Take the right diet for weight loss

#3: Exercise

#4: Change your mental attitude.

Everything we will discuss in the subsequent chapters will somehow relate to these four points.

The Right Way To Lose Weight

It is natural for anyone wanting to lose weight to try to lose it very quickly. But research has proven that people who do it gradually and steadily, are more likely to maintain their weight in the long run. Healthy weight loss is much more than a program or diet. It is about a progressive lifestyle that incorporates long-term changes in exercise habits and daily eating. Ideally, in order to lose weight, you need to burn more calories than you eat.

One pound (of the human body) is equivalent to about 3500 calories. As such, you have to lower your caloric intake by 500 to 1000 calories per day in order to shade approximately one to two pounds per week. Different people require different amounts of energy (energy in this case is measured in calories).

The basic rule of losing weight is to push your body to start burning stored fat-you don't want it to start losing muscle mass. Before you get started, you should understand how many calories you need daily depending on your activity level so that you can actually work towards consuming less calories to push your body to a calorie deficit condition whereby it is forced to burn stored fat. Here is a calculator to help you determine your daily calorie requirement. Here is another calculator to help you in the process of losing weight.

When you achieve a healthy weight by relying on physical activity and healthy eating for most of the days of the week, you have a better chance of maintaining the weight for the long term. It is not easy to lose weight – it takes commitment. The good news is that no matter how much weight you want to lose, even a subtle weight lose, of say, 5 – 10 percent of your overall body weight is more likely to produce healthy results, e.g. reduction in blood cholesterol, blood pressure, and blood sugar level.

For instance, if you weigh 190 pounds, a five percent weight loss would bring your weight down to 180.5 pounds. While you may still be in the "overweight" or "obese" category, this subtle weight loss can reduce your risk factors for chronic diseases associated with obesity. Therefore, even if the ultimate goal seems too large, consider it a journey, rather than a final destination. We are going to discover new eating and exercise habits that will help you live a healthier lifestyle. These new habits will also go a long way towards helping you maintain a healthy weight over time. As we've already discussed, maintaining a healthy weight is more likely to come with a variety of other benefits. You will experience improvement in your energy levels, general mood, physical mobility, and self confidence.

The first step to sustainable weight loss is to get rid of the toxins in the body. I already talked about how my journey to sustainable weight loss started. You too can start with the body cleanse.

Cleanse/Detoxify Your Body

Basically, natural cleansing means flushing out accumulated toxins and wastes from your body, leaving you feeling better than ever before. Detoxification is simply the process of cleaning blood and entails removal of impurities from the blood in the liver (toxins are often processed in the liver for elimination). Other channels of toxin removal include the skin, intestines, lymph, lungs, and kidneys.

There are several natural ways you can cleanse and detoxify your system. For instance, including specific natural rituals coupled with making food, drink and lifestyle choices can actually help you cleanse your body and sustain that over time. With a detox program, you can help your body's natural cleansing process through:

>Enhancing the circulation of blood

>Resting organs through fasting

>Enhancing elimination through the skin, kidneys and intestines

>Stimulating the liver to make it drive toxins from the body

>Refueling your body with healthy nutrients

Alkalizing the body is one of the best strategies you can use to detoxify the body. Actually, many of the detox methods that you will see in this book revolve around alkalizing the body. Let's first understand the process of alkalizing the body.

Alkalize your body

Our bodies work really hard to process the foods we eat and drink. Give your body a break sometimes, even if it means changing what you drink for a day. Take a day off and don't drink anything but water, preferably warm water with lemon. Your goal is to get your body to an alkaline state. The quickest and most convenient way to alkalize the body is lemon.

Technically, lemon is an acid before you consume it, but once your body starts processing it, it turns alkaline. The correct pH level for normal human blood is above 7.0, at which it is very hard for you to get sick. When it gets below 7.0, you become susceptible to a variety of diseases. One of our daily goals when it comes to good health is to keep a neutral PH level. When you have a heartburn, gas, or a bloated stomach, it's because your body is in an acidic state. No one should be taking antacids on a regular basis. That's not normal. With this new lifestyle change, I never get any of the above. There are many alkaline foods; check the list in the back of the book. Let's first discuss some few methods through which you can detoxify your body.

Drink plenty of water

One of the most important things you need to do when trying to naturally cleanse your body is to increase your water intake. You should generally aim to drink at least eight glasses of water, or 2 quarts throughout the day. The first step in increasing your water intake is to drink a glass the first thing when you wake up in the morning, and after every snack or meal you take. Other ways you can add water to your body is to eat fruits and veggies with a high concentration of water, such as tomatoes, cucumber, strawberries, and watermelon. Water is significant in the detoxification process in the following ways:

*Water flushes out impurities and toxins from your body by helping your bowel and kidneys to maintain their normal functions of eliminating waste.

*Water also plays a major role in keeping the skin looking young and healthy, clearing the complexion and preventing wrinkles.

*Water preserved in bottles or copper vessels is cleansed and purified due to copper's antibacterial properties.

Eat more fiber

Fiber is the most important nutrient in maintaining proper digestion and is therefore, a fantastic natural cleanser. Including more fiber in your diet helps your body rid itself of preservatives, toxins and other harmful waste materials that have accumulated in the digestive tract over time. Fiber works to cleanse your body by triggering regular bowel movements thus leaving you feeling healthy and light, as opposed to sluggish and bloated. The best natural sources include rice, pasta, whole grain cereals, fresh fruit and vegetables, almonds, lentils and beans.

Avoid alcohol and caffeine

As far as the cleansing process is concerned, alcohol and caffeine are two substances that you should avoid as much as possible. The toxins contained in these substances can impair both the liver and kidney function, which can subsequently diminish your body's ability to cleanse itself naturally. When this happens, it can increase your risk for obesity and diabetes.

During the growing process, coffee is often exposed to pesticides and herbicides. Coffee also has no proven health benefits on the body, and can contribute to dehydration. If you need something to stimulate you in the morning, green tea is a much better choice because it contains a small amount of caffeine, as well as healthy antioxidants.

Alcohol, on the other hand, especially dark liquors such as red wine, rum and whiskey, contain toxins called congeners that are formed as a byproduct of the fermentation process. Apart from these congeners, alcohol also releases a toxic substance called acetaldehyde after it metabolizes in the body.

Restrict your simple carbohydrate intake

Simple carbohydrates such as white rice, pasta and bread are essentially deficient in vitamins, nutrients, and any other substances that are good for your body. While it is true that they will make you feel full at first, they are also accompanied by a spike and fall in your blood sugar, which is hazardous for your energy levels, and overall health. Simple carbohydrates are also often filled with preservatives that can accumulate in your system, resulting in the development of toxins. To counter this problem, turn to complex carbohydrates and more high fiber whole grain foods, like those found in starchy vegetables such as potatoes, pastas & cereals, wholegrain breads, legumes and brown rice. Complex carbohydrates have far much better benefits on the digestive system, and can help you clear out the accumulated preservatives and toxins.

Eat more super foods

While it is generally advisable to restrict your intake of processed foods during the cleansing process, you need to eat as much super foods as possible. These are specific foods with extraordinary health benefits, one of them being helping your body to speed up the cleansing process. The four most beneficial super foods are listed below, but others include wild rice, papaya, carrots, Brussels Sprouts, celery, watercress, apples and blueberries.

*Garlic: There are several significant health benefits of garlic, but perhaps the most important one is its ability to enhance liver function by helping in the production of enzymes that help the liver to eliminate toxins from your body. Garlic also contains two substances referred to as selenium and allicin, which have been found to be beneficial in cleansing the liver.

*Beets: Bright red beets contain anti-inflammatory, antioxidant and detoxifying properties because of their high levels of betalain, the natural pigment that gives these super foods their vibrant color. Keep in mind that beets tend to lose their most important health benefits when cooked, so the best way to get the most out of them is to eat them raw.

*Kale: This is a very healthy leafy green vegetable with significant cleansing properties. Kale, as well as other greens such as cabbage, is slightly alkaline. It therefore has the ability to neutralize sugars and other toxins before they are flushed out of your body. As such, kale helps to maintain your blood in its natural, slightly alkaline state.

*Lemon: Lemon, as well as other citrus fruits such as lime and grapefruit, are widely recognized to be one of the best natural cleansers in the world. This is probably why lemons are included in many body-flush and juice cleanse recipes. Lemons are packed with citric acid that has the ability to neutralize accumulated toxins in the body, enabling them to be flushed out through urine. As a general rule of thumb, make a point of squeezing some lemon juice in a glass of water the first thing when you wake up in the morning, or just eat a grapefruit for breakfast.

Drink herbal teas

A great way to increase your fluid intake while also enjoying the numerous natural cleansing benefits of natural herbs and roots provided by Mother Nature is to engage in herbal teas. Here are some of the most beneficial teas you can drink:

*Dandelion tea: Dandelion tea works to cleanse the body by stimulating the liver, kidneys and gall bladder, thus reducing water retention and allowing your body to flush out impurities faster. It is also believed to help stabilize blood sugar levels, as well as boosting the immune system. You can find dandelion tea in most health food stores, but you can also make your own by boiling fresh dandelions in water.

*Licorice tea: Licorice is a substance that has several health benefits. However, as an internal cleanser, it helps to enhance liver function while acting as a mild laxative at the same time thus aiding to clear the bowels by getting rid of accumulated waste. You can find licorice tea in health food stores, but you can also boil the root in a pint of water to prepare your own. Be aware that licorice tea may not be compatible with people with high blood pressure, so it is advisable to consult your doctor before engaging.

*Burdock tea: This root has been used for centuries in natural remedies, and its superior health benefits are still acknowledged today. It is a natural blood purifier that helps to cleanse and detoxify the blood, eliminating any accumulated impurities. It also stimulates the production of urine, and cleanses the intestinal tract to help flush out from the system. It also helps to protect and repair the liver, which can go a long way to counter the effects of alcohol. You can purchase burdock tea or boil a small amount of the root in water.

Eat organic produce

Go for organically grown fruits and vegetables, as well as organically produced meat and dairy products. While organic produce might be expensive, it does not contain synthetic pesticides and fertilizers. It also uses a small amount of antibiotics and growth hormones. When you limit yourself to organically produced foods, you also limit your body's exposure to the toxic chemicals contained in these pesticides and other substances involved in the production of non-organic foods.

Quit smoking

One of the worst things you can do to include toxins in your body is smoking. Apart from nicotine, most commercial cigarettes contain more than 4000 other toxic chemicals. Even if you quit smoking, these toxins will remain in your system for some time. As such, smoking is one of the first things that you need to do if you are trying to detox your body naturally. Your body can flush out these toxins gradually on its own, but you can accelerate the process by drinking plenty of water, getting plenty of exercise, and eating healthy, and fiber rich foods.

Take apple cider vinegar

Apple cider vinegar is a product obtained from the fermentation of apples. In this process, the sugars contained in the apples are broken down and turned to alcohol by yeast and bacteria. If the process continues further, it turns to vinegar. Most people have been using apple cider vinegar to make dressing salads and pickles. Taking apple cider vinegar can give you the much needed boost to your weight loss process. However, keep in mind that it tends to work gradually, and not rapidly. It has two benefits, namely: giving your body enough time to adjust to the weight loss, and ensuring that the pounds you have lost do not bounce back.

*Apple cider vinegar has organic acids and enzymes, which increase the rate of metabolism, thereby speeding up the process of burning fat in your body. Vinegar is rich in acetic acid, which helps extract iron from the food you eat, as well as availing it to building blocks for oxygen carrying hemoglobin. This in turn helps in enhancing metabolism. With enhanced metabolism, it becomes a lot easier to lose weight.

*It makes you feel satiated, which means you will eat less and lose weight faster. It also retains water, making you feel and look thinner. Additionally, it helps burn fat in your body by enhancing the slow release of glucose into your bloodstream, as opposed to storing it. This basically makes you feel fuller for longer by suppressing your hunger.

*It reduces water retention in your body, and hydrates you by freshening your body.

*It is also rich in fiber and potassium, which lower blood sugar levels, which in turn help in weight loss.

*ACV also contains high amounts of pectin, potash, minerals, enzymes, vitamins, and acids such as propionic acid, alcoholic acid, amino acids, acetic acid, and other acids that make this vinegar the ideal diet supplement. All these properties will help speed up the rate of metabolism, enabling you to lose weight quickly without having to sacrifice on any essential nutrients in your body.

*It also enhances proper digestion by helping get rid of stored waste in the colon and intestines, which means fat is not stored in your body, and you do not gain weight.

*This vinegar also helps to eliminate harmful toxins from your body, as well as burning calories to help you shed the excess weight.

*Apple cider vinegar is also very effective in lowering cholesterol levels, as well as making you feel healthy and energetic in general.

*It is packed with natural antiseptic and antibiotic properties, which are effective in fighting germs and bacteria.

Use honey

What if someone told you that you could fit into that dressing you have always admired by Christmas by simply eating a teaspoon of honey each night before you go to bed? The deal seems too good to be true, but this is a new revolutionary and scientifically backed way of getting slim.

Honey has been shown to trigger metabolic changes that ascertain you won't succumb to sugar cravings or burn fat when sleeping. Honey is considered a more natural sweetener as opposed to regular white sugar. Studies have also shown that it also contains anti microbial, anti inflammatory and antioxidant effects, and can help in healing. However, before you reach for that jar of honey, be aware that there are other factors to consider.

-When losing weight, the key is to achieve a calorie deficit, which essentially means consuming fewer calories than you burn. As such, you have to ensure that anything you eat fits into your daily calorie allowance. There are approximately twenty-one calories in a teaspoon of honey. The daily calorie allowance for most women is basically around 1600 to 2400 calories to maintain weight, while for most men it is between 2000 and 3000 calories.

In order to lose weight, you need to eat slightly less than this, which means that whatever amount of honey you eat needs to fit into your calorie goal.

Honey can serve as a natural hunger suppressant thus making it an ideal weight loss solution. Taking a drink of honey before going to bed can help your body burn calories, repair and stop sugar cravings. As a general rule of thumb, ensure that you cut out on junk food, eat more fresh fruit and vegetables, lean proteins, and switch from processed to unrefined carbohydrates.

Avoid environmental toxins

This can be tricky, especially since our air today is so polluted, and there is a pervasive overuse of chemicals in virtually every aspect of our life. Whenever you can, you should try as much as possible to surround yourself with clean fresh air, and avoid breathing in factory smoke and city smog. If you can, escape to the seaside or countryside for the weekend to clear the city air from your lungs. In addition, avoid as much as possible breathing in second hand smoke and clean your home with natural cleaning products to avoid unnecessary exposure to toxic chemicals. Get out of the house and take a walk along the lake or in the park. It enhances your mind and body's functioning, and helps you stay fit as well.

Exercise

One of the most healthy and natural ways to cleanse your body is by doing regular exercise. Exercise gets the body moving, and also keeps it functioning at full capacity. It will also enhance your weight loss campaign, thus eliminating the toxins that have accumulated in your fat cells over the years. Toxins are also eliminated from your body through perspiration, which is the most natural way to cleanse the body. Try to incorporate 4 or 5 half hour sessions of moderate to high intensity exercise into your routine – anything from dancing, climbing, swimming or running. You will feel healthier and happier in no time.

Get more sleep

Technically, sleep is not responsible for cleansing the body by itself, but it is nonetheless crucial for living a healthy life and maintaining normal body function. Sleep is necessary for your body to recover and repair itself after the strains and stresses of daily life. Getting seven to eight hours of sleep as recommended by doctors helps your body prepare for the activities of the next day, providing you with more energy for exercise and other activities. You also need quality sleep for a healthy immune system, without which your body would not be able to deal with harmful toxins, bacteria and viruses it is consistently bombarded with. Sleep deprivation can put you at a higher risk of developing obesity, diabetes, high blood pressure, kidney disease, and heart disease.

Manage your stress

Stress can go a long way towards creating a negative impact on your overall health because it hinders the production of good hormones, and impairs your body from performing at its optimum level. The absence of these hormones means that your body retains toxins that in turn cause you to feel tired and depressed. This subsequently leads to further weight gain, as well as unhealthy lifestyle choices. You can encourage the production of good hormones by keeping your stress levels to a minimum. If you have a busy life and are still trying to reduce your stress levels, yoga and meditation are excellent choices. When you focus only on your breathing, you can clean and cleanse your mind which in turn, will have a positive impact on your body.

Try fasting for a day or two

One popular way to cleanse the body is through fasting, which involves cutting out or limiting your body's intake of food severely while flushing out toxins from your system with high volumes of liquid. The point is to make your body start afresh while cleansed and renewed.

Specific Cleanses
Try the lemonade cleanse

This is one of the most popular cleanses in the world, thanks to numerous celebrity advocates. This cleanse involves making a drink out of lemon juice, water, cayenne pepper and maple syrup, and then consuming it exclusively for 3 to 10 days. The work of this cleanse is to help you flush out toxins from your system, while also helping in weight loss. You can make a glass of lemonade by mixing half a teaspoon of organic maple syrup, 4 tablespoons of freshly squeezed lemon juice, and a teaspoon of cayenne pepper into a 10 ounce glass of water. Four to five times of this quantity is enough to last you the whole day. However, just keep in mind that medical experts do not support this cleanse because it creates a serious nutrient and calorie deficit that can lead to a negative effect on your health.

Try the ginger and apple cleanse

This is a less intense version of the previous lemonade cleanse. You only need to take it once per week, and you can also accompany it with some light and healthy snacks. This recipe includes psyllium husk, in addition to the ginger and apple. Psyllium husk is a type of dietary fiber that is believed to effectively bind together waste material, making it easier for your system to flush them out. You can prepare the juice cleanse by combining 8 ounces of organic or freshly pressed apples with a teaspoon of ground psyllium husk and ginger. Blend at a low speed or mix well with a spoon. After taking this mixture, you need to drink plenty of water throughout the day, because this will help keep your digestive system moving.

Do a salt water flush

This is another popular but rather unpleasant way to rid your system of accumulated waste and toxins. Salt is a natural disinfectant that efficiently flushes out the whole intestinal tract. In fact, because of the effectiveness of this process, it is often used as a cheaper alternative to the costly colonic irrigation procedures. You are basically supposed to drink a glass of water on an empty stomach, and then wait for an hour or so as the solution flushes your bowels out, leading to numerous eliminations. You can prepare the salt solution by dissolving 2 teaspoons of non-ionized, unrefined sea salt into 1 quart of purified, lukewarm water. Make a point of drinking the solution when you wake up in the morning, and then lie on your side for thirty minutes. This helps the salt water to pass into the small intestine. When this happens, you will feel the urge to eliminate, so be sure to stay near a bathroom. Keep in mind that intense diarrhea and vomiting are common after a salt water flush.

After cleansing your body, the next thing you should do is to embrace different strategies to help you lose weight. Unlike the popular belief that all you have to do is to eat less food, you need to realize that you have to eat well for your blood type. Let's discuss that in the next chapter.

Eat Right For Your Blood Type

If you didn't know yet, you should understand that you must eat right for your blood type. I learnt about the blood type diet when I read about Peter J. D'Adamo's study that if you are of blood type O, you have to eat foods that are best suited for blood type O. The same applies to blood type A, B and AB. Food reacts chemically based on the blood type. This is especially because of the effect of proteins referred to as Lectins that become active when they interact with your blood type. Essentially, eating foods best suited for a specific blood type will result to efficient digestion, improved energy, increased immunity and weight loss just to mention a few of the effects. If you don't take the right foods (especially if you are blood groups A and O), you are likely to experience such problems like bloating and food intolerance issues. The walls of the stomach and the intestines are usually lined with sensitive receptors that interact with lectin. Although a single reaction might not be much of a problem, continuing reaction could result to dire problems including deterioration of health, weight gain, and loss of energy. Well, we all know all that spells WEIGHT GAIN because when you don't have energy or are sick, you are likely to feel sluggish such that you don't want to engage in any physical activity, which means you are likely to start having lots of calorie surpluses resulting to weight gain. I will be pretty straight forward on what to eat for different blood groups to help you in making informed food choices by removing targeted foods and then replacing them with foods that are more suitable for your blood type. With that, you are likely to start experiencing improved energy and weight loss.

Type A blood

Ideally, you should eat a meat free diet that is based on vegetables and fruits, legumes and beans, whole grains (fresh and organic). If you have this blood type, you are likely to have a sensitive immune system. A blood type can be summarized as follows:

A= Agrarian

*Vegetarian diet, has a very sensitive digestive tract, responds well to stress with calming actions and even gentle exercise, adapts quite well to settled environmental and dietary conditions, has a tolerant immune system and requires agrarian diet in order to stay lean and productive.

Type B blood

You should avoid wheat, lentils, corn, sesame seeds, peanuts, tomatoes and buckwheat. You should also avoid or minimize your intake of chicken. Instead, you should take more green vegetables, low fat dairy, selected meats and eggs. Here is a quick summary of B.

B= Nomadic

Blood type B has a tolerant digestive system, is best suited for low fat dairy, produce and meat, requires moderate exercise, responds well to stress through creativity and requires balance between physical and mental activity in order to stay lean and sharp. You should avoid wheat. This blood type can tolerate the most flexible dietary choices.

Type AB blood

In this case, you should take more of green vegetables, dairy, seafood, and tofu. Since you are likely to have low stomach acid, you should avoid cured or smoked meats, alcohol and caffeine. Here is a quick summary for Blood type AB.

AB=Modern

This blood type should avoid beef, pork and chicken, has a highly sensitive digestive tract, and responds well to stress spiritually with creative energy and physical activity.

Type O blood

You should take a high protein diet that is high in fish, poultry, lean meat, light grains, dairy, vegetables and beans. You should also take more supplements to help solve different tummy problems that you are likely to have. The blood type is intolerant to environmental and dietary adaptations. This blood type requires an efficient metabolism in order to stay energetic and lean. The best method for coping with stress is through vigorous exercise.

As for physical exercise, you should also remember that specific exercises are ideal for different blood types. For instance, if you are type A, you should do tai chi or yoga. On the other hand, if you are type O, you should try vigorous aerobic exercises such as biking and jogging.

It is also important to note that you should insist on taking more of raw foods as opposed to cooked foods if you really want to keep your body alkaline, detoxify and lose weight. Let's take a look at why raw foods are better than cooked foods.

Raw foods Vs Cooked foods

Eating raw food brings more nutritional benefits than cooked foods. Well, although cooked food is likely to taste delicious, it might not actually be good for you. Actually, it might be killing you slowly. In a nutshell, cooking kills essential nutrients which essentially means that when you eat cooked food, you are eating food that is stripped off of its nutrients. The enzymes, pytonutrients, minerals, fiber, essential fats, vitamins and proteins are destroyed when you cook food. As such, if cooking is known to destroy all essential nutrients that we need in order to stay healthy, eating raw food gives us all these benefits. When I embraced raw food diet, I have noticed that I have more energy and have greater mental focus. I also don't have to worry about acid reflux, aches, dissipate and other problems because I feed my body with what it needs in order to thrive and not just what it needs to survive.

You should mix this up with the herbs in order to boost your immune system, increase metabolism and achieve many more benefits. Some common herbs you should try for weight loss, stress relief and detoxification include:

Herbs for detox: Dandelion, aloe vera, milk thistle, cilantro, wormwood, turmeric, ginger, eucalyptus etc.

Herbs for weight loss: green tea, fish oil, ginseng, hibiscus tea, guggul, yerba mate, pu-erh tea, grape fruit etc.

Herbs for stress relief: passion flower, kava kava, St. John's wort, licorice root, lavender etc.

Please note that each herb requires a unique usage approach. As such, you should ensure that you learn about each herb before using it.

Here is a list of alkalizing foods that you should take in more quantities if you want to stay healthy, detoxify, have more energy and lose weight.

ALKALIZING VEGETABLES
Cauliflower
Celery
Chard Greens
Chlorella
Pumpkin
Radishes
Rutabaga
Collard Greens
Cucumber
Parsnips (high glycemic)
Peas
Peppers
Mushrooms
Mustard Greens
Nightshade Veggies
Onions
Sprouts
Sweet Potatoes
Tomatoes
Watercress
Wheat Grass
Sea Veggies
Spinach, green
Spirulina
Wild Greens
Alfalfa
Barley Grass
Beet Greens
Beets
Broccoli
Cabbage
Carrot
Dandelions
Dulce
Edible Flowers
Eggplant
Fermented Veggies
Garlic
Green Beans
Green Peas
Kale
Kohlrabi
Lettuce

ALKALIZING ORIENTAL VEGETABLES
Daikon
Dandelion Root
Nori
Reishi
Kombu
Maitake
Shitake
Umeboshi
Wakame

ALKALIZING FRUITS
Honeydew Melon
Lemon
Lime
Muskmelons
Berries
Blackberries
Cantaloupe
Cherries, sour
Raisins
Raspberries
Rhubarb
Strawberries
Grapes
Grapefruit
Coconut, fresh
Currants
Dates, dried
Figs, dried
Nectarine
Orange
Peach
Pear
Pineapple
Tomato
Tropical Fruits
Umeboshi Plums
Watermelon
Tangerine
Apple
Apricot
Avocado
Banana (high glycemic)

ALKALIZING SWEETENERS
Stevia

ALKALIZING SPICES & SEASONINGS
Sea Salt
Tamari
Herbs (all)
Ginger
Chili Pepper
Cinnamon
Curry
Miso
Mustard

ALKALIZING OTHER
Fresh Fruit Juice
Green Juices
Lecithin Granules
Mineral Water
Alkaline Antioxidant Water
Apple Cider Vinegar
Bee Pollen
Soured Dairy Products
Veggie Juices
Molasses, blackstrap
Probiotic Cultures

ALKALIZING MINERALS
Magnesium: pH 9
Potassium: pH 14
Sodium: pH 14
Calcium: pH 12
Cesium: pH 14

Please note that a food's acid forming or alkaline tendency in your body has completely nothing to do with the natural pH level of the food itself. That's why you will see lemon being alkalizing despite it being acidic in its natural form. You should also be aware of the acid forming foods so that you can reduce their intake. Here is a list of the acid forming foods just to help you understand what foods you should avoid.

ACIDIFYING GRAINS, GRAIN PRODUCTS
Rice Cakes
Rye
Spaghetti
Spelt
Wheat Germ
Wheat
Noodles
Oatmeal
Oats (rolled)
Kamut
Macaroni
Quinoa
Rice (all)
Cornstarch
Crackers, soda
Flour, wheat
Flour, white
Hemp Seed Flour
Bran, wheat
Bread
Corn
Amaranth
Barley
Bran, oat

ACIDIFYING ALCOHOL
Beer
Wine
Hard Liquor
Spirits

ACIDIFYING DRUGS & CHEMICALS
Herbicides
Pesticides
Drugs, Psychedelic
Tobacco
Aspirin
Chemicals
Drugs, Medicinal

ACIDIFYING VEGETABLES
Winter Squash
Olives
Corn
Lentils

ACIDIFYING FRUITS
Cranberries
Currants
Blueberries
Plums**
Prunes**
Canned or Glazed Fruits

ACIDIFYING DAIRY
Cheese, Processed
Ice Cream
Ice Milk
Butter
Cheese

ACIDIFYING ANIMAL PROTEIN
Rabbit
Salmon
Sardines
Sausage
Scallops
Corned Beef
Fish
Haddock
Tuna
Turkey
Veal
Venison
Pike
Pork
Lamb
Lobster
Mussels
Organ Meats
Oyster
Shellfish
Shrimp
Bacon
Beef
Carp
Clams
Cod

ACIDIFYING BEANS & LEGUMES
Lentils
Pinto Beans
White Beans
Almond Milk
Kidney Beans
Red Beans
Green Peas
Chick Peas
Rice Milk
Soy Beans
Soy Milk
Black Beans

ACIDIFYING NUTS & BUTTERS
Pecans
Tahini
Peanuts
Walnuts
Cashews
Legumes
Peanut Butter

ACIDIFYING SWEETENERS
Carob
Corn Syrup
Sugar

ACIDIFYING OTHER FOODS
Catsup
Cocoa
Soft Drinks
Vinegar
Coffee
Mustard
Pepper

ACIDIFYING JUNK FOOD
Beer: pH 2.5
Coca-Cola: pH 2
Coffee: pH 4

Conclusion

Even as you embrace everything you have learnt throughout the book, I will insist on combining this with physical exercise. Aim for at least 4 times of physical activity (it could be light intensity or high intensity exercise) if you really want sustainable weight loss. Your health is also likely to improve over time when you embrace regular exercise. For instance, you are likely to reduce your likelihood of suffering from cardiovascular diseases and many others. Being healthy and losing weight is a holistic process; you cannot just avoid one thing and consider it okay. Actually, failure to do everything is likely to result to problems.